GALVESTON

DIET

By

PULL ROSE ALEXANDRA

Disclaimer

TABLE OF CONTENT

INTRODUCTION

The Galveston Diet has become a well-known and talked-about method for controlling weight and improving general health. This nutritional plan was created by board-certified OB-GYN Dr. Mary Claire Haver, who is passionate about women's health. It specifically targets the obstacles that women have on their path to wellbeing.

As we explore the nuances of the Galveston Diet, it becomes clear that its basis is a sophisticated understanding of hormonal impacts and the unique requirements of the female body, in addition to sound nutritional principles. Fundamentally, the goal of the Galveston Diet is to promote hormonal balance, especially for women who are approaching or have reached menopause. Dr. Haver is aware of the significant effects that changes in hormones may have on a woman's metabolism, energy levels, and ability to regulate her weight at different stages of life.

The diet places a strong emphasis on nutrient-dense, whole foods that support hormonal balance in an effort to lessen these consequences. The Galveston Diet's emphasis on anti-inflammatory foods is one of its main tenets. Dr. Haver emphasizes how hormone abnormalities and weight gain are only two health problems that are exacerbated by chronic inflammation.

The diet promotes foods that have anti-inflammatory qualities, such as berries, leafy greens, and fatty fish, in an effort to establish an internal environment that promotes general well-being. Additionally, the Galveston Diet emphasizes the need to balance macronutrients—carbs, fats, and proteins.

In contrast to certain fad diets that stigmatize whole food categories, this strategy acknowledges the significance of every macronutrient in maintaining optimum health. Foods high in protein aid in maintaining muscular mass, which is necessary for metabolism and general strength. Nutritious fats, including those in avocados and olive oil, help with satiety and hormonal support. Whole grains and vegetables are good sources of complex carbs, which provide sustained energy and vital nutrients.

The Galveston Diet stands out because it recognizes the particular hormonal difficulties that women have as they age. Progesterone, testosterone, and estrogen are examples of hormones that are important for metabolism and body composition. Women often suffer changes in fat distribution, an increase in belly fat, and a reduced metabolism after menopause due to these hormone fluctuations.

This knowledge is included in the structure of the Galveston Diet, which customizes food recommendations to promote hormonal balance and lessen the impact of these shifts. The Galveston Diet promotes intermittent fasting as an adjunctive tactic in addition to dietary recommendations.

Research indicates that intermittent fasting, which alternates between eating and fasting times, may provide a number of health advantages, including better metabolic health and weight control. The Galveston Diet adheres to the idea of creating a strategy that complements the lifestyle of its practitioners by including intermittent fasting in a sustainable and controllable manner. The Galveston Diet includes more than just nutrition; it's a whole-person approach to wellness. Recognizing the importance of exercise in preserving muscle mass, promoting cardiovascular health, and improving general well-being, it promotes regular physical activity.

The Galveston Diet differs from other restrictive diet regimens in that it emphasizes a holistic lifestyle approach. Dr. Haver takes a well-rounded, evidence-based approach to her approach, drawing on both scientific research and her clinical expertise. The Galveston Diet recognizes the uniqueness of every woman's health journey rather than offering a one-size-fits-all answer.

This customized component is essential because it acknowledges the important roles that genetics, lifestyle, and medical history play in determining dietary requirements and reactions. Success stories and testimonies to the Galveston Diet's increasing popularity underscore its beneficial effects on women's lives. Many report increased vigor, happiness, and energy levels in addition to weight reduction. The diet's attraction stems from its emphasis on long-term sustainability, which encourages a mental shift away from temporary remedies and toward long-term lifestyle adjustments.

CHAPTER ONE

YOUR WANTS AND PHYSIQUE ARE EVOLVING.

I am a machine learning model, not a real being with shifting needs. I can, however, assist you in investigating the idea of shifting wants and bodies within the framework of human experiences. From birth to old age, the human body experiences a great deal of change. These alterations affect not only the physical body but also the emotional, social, and psychological domains. Living a happy and healthy life requires recognizing these changes and learning to embrace them.

The human body experiences fast growth and development throughout infancy. Newborns go from being completely dependent on others to being able to manage their fundamental motor abilities. The body's demands change as it gets older, moving from basic nutrition to more intricate mental and emotional stimulation. Childhood is a time of discovery and learning, during which the body learns to become more skilled at different tasks.

During this time, education, social connection, and the growth of emotional intelligence are among the shifting demands. Hormonal changes brought about by puberty cause major physical changes that affect the person's view of themselves as well as their physique. Adolescence is a crucial time when people start to define their identities and establish their individuality. The body's evolving demands include an emphasis on developing a sense of purpose, self-expression, and interpersonal interactions. Peer influence is quite important at this point in forming preferences and actions.

As one approaches maturity, more physiological and psychological changes occur. When one's physical state reaches its pinnacle, attention often turns to one's work, relationships, and stability. People start to want autonomy more and more when they try to make decisions on their own. When people get older, their bodies gradually lose some of their physical capacities. In addition to possible changes in bone density and muscle mass, metabolism slows down. Maintaining one's health, having a stable profession, and taking care of one's family are often among the shifting requirements at this time. People could also reassess their objectives in life and take up new pastimes or interests. More noticeable physical changes occur in later life, often coupled with health issues.

There might be a decline in sensory perception and an increased susceptibility to diseases. During this stage, the requirements that change most often center on health care, company, and a feeling of legacy. Keeping up social ties and thinking back on past experiences become essential elements of wellbeing. It is impossible to overestimate the significance of mental and emotional health throughout these different phases of life. Finding purpose in every stage of life and adjusting to shifting circumstances are mostly dependent on the intellect. Navigating the difficulties brought on by a changing body and changing requirements requires the development of resilience and coping skills. In summary, both physically and emotionally, the human experience is a journey marked by constant change.

To adjust to these modifications, one must recognize and comprehend the changing demands at various phases of life. Every stage of life offers new chances and challenges for development, whether it is the unbounded energy of childhood, the self-discovery of adolescence, the need for stability in maturity, or introspection in old age. A more contented and significant existence may be achieved by accepting these adjustments and tackling them with optimism.

CHAPTER TWO

GAINING CONTROL OF YOUR HORMONES

It's essential to comprehend and control your hormones for general wellbeing. Hormones are chemical messengers that are essential to many body processes; they affect mood, energy levels, metabolism, and reproductive health, among other things. Hormonal equilibrium is necessary to preserve both physical and mental well-being. This thorough guide will assist you in managing your hormones.

1. Know Your Hormones: To start, educate yourself on the main hormones that control various aspects of your health. Cortisol, insulin, thyroid hormones, progesterone, estrogen, testosterone, and other hormones are among them. Every hormone has a distinct purpose, and any imbalance in any one of them might result in a number of health problems.

2. Balanced Diet: Hormone control is greatly influenced by nutrition. It is crucial to have a diet that is well-balanced and rich in different nutrients. Make sure you're receiving enough vitamins, minerals, healthy fats, and proteins. Fish and flaxseeds are good sources of omega-3 fatty acids, which are especially helpful for hormone synthesis.

3. Handle stress: Prolonged stress may upset the equilibrium of hormones, especially by raising cortisol levels. Include stress-relieving

activities in your routine, such as yoga, deep breathing techniques, or meditation. Additionally, getting enough sleep is essential because it controls hormones like cortisol.

4. Frequent Exercise: Exercise is essential for the health of your hormones. Exercise increases metabolism, balances sex hormones, and helps control insulin. For general health and well-being, try to include both strength and cardio training.

5. Enough sleep: Hormone synthesis and control depend on getting a good night's sleep. Sleep deprivation may mess with the ratios of hormones like ghrelin and leptin, which can impact metabolism and hunger. Aim for seven to nine hours of good sleep every night.

6. Keep a Healthy Weight: Hormonal equilibrium may be affected by being overweight or underweight. For general hormonal health, it is essential to reach and maintain a healthy weight via a balanced diet and frequent exercise.

7. Hormone Disruptors: Be cautious when you come into contact with things that might interfere with hormones' ability to work normally. These include some of the compounds included in insecticides, plastics, and several personal hygiene items. Whenever feasible, use natural and organic goods.

8. Keep Yourself Hydrated: Hormone control depends on being well hydrated. Water facilitates many physiological functions and aids in the movement of hormones throughout the body. Make it a daily goal to consume enough water.

9. Frequent Check-ups: Make an appointment with your healthcare practitioner on a frequent basis to have your hormone levels checked. Blood testing may provide important information about your hormonal health and aid in the early detection of any abnormalities or problems.

10. Hormone Replacement Therapy (HRT): Medical intervention may be necessary in some circumstances due to hormonal abnormalities. Restoring hormonal equilibrium with hormone replacement therapy under the supervision of a medical expert may be successful. This is especially important for diseases like hypothyroidism and menopause.

11. Hormones and Birth Control: It's important for those taking hormonal contraceptives to be aware of the possible effects on hormonal balance. To make an educated choice, go over alternatives and possible side effects with your healthcare professional.

12. Recognize Menstrual Health: For those who have monthly periods, being aware of and monitoring their menstrual health may provide important insights regarding changes in hormone levels. Calendars and

apps may be used to anticipate and control hormonal shifts that occur throughout the menstrual cycle.

13. Hormones and Mental Health: An important relationship exists between hormones and mental health. Anxiety, melancholy, and mood swings may all be attributed to imbalances. Seek expert assistance to treat both the psychological and hormonal components of chronic mental health disorders.

14. Hormones and Aging: Hormone levels normally change with aging. It's essential for healthy aging to recognize these changes and modify your lifestyle to meet your changing hormonal demands. Stress reduction, a healthy diet, and regular exercise become even more important.

15. Seek Professional Guidance: Speak with a healthcare provider if you feel that you may have a hormone imbalance or if you are exhibiting symptoms like weight gain, exhaustion, or irregular menstruation periods. They may carry out pertinent testing and provide you with tailored advice depending on your particular health profile.

CHAPTER THREE:

GET READY TO TRANSFORM YOUR LIFE

Starting a path to transform your life takes careful planning and a dedication to personal development. This article examines the necessary actions and changes in perspective to guarantee a transition that is effective. Body:

1. Self-Reflection: To start, consider your present circumstances and note your advantages, disadvantages, and potential growth areas. This self-examination lays the groundwork for significant transformation.

2. Establish Your Objectives: Clearly state your immediate and long-term objectives. Creating SMART (specific, measurable, attainable, relevant, and time-bound) goals gives your change a path forward.

3. Make a strategy: Come up with a detailed strategy that outlines the actions required to accomplish your objectives. Divide more ambitious goals into more doable activities, and set benchmarks to monitor your progress.

4. Create a Support System: Assemble a group of people who will help you develop and who are great influences in your life. Strong support networks may provide direction, inspiration, and responsibility.

5. Educate yourself: Personal growth requires ongoing learning. Make time to learn new skills, keep up with current events, and pursue information related to your objectives.

6. Accept Change: Adapting to change frequently means moving outside of your comfort zone. Accept pain as a sign of development and keep an open mind to novel, boundary-pushing events.

7. Create Healthy Habits: Form routines that support your mental, emotional, and physical health. This may include mindfulness exercises, a healthy diet, enough sleep, and frequent exercise.

8. Effective Time Management: Time is an important resource. Acquire the skills necessary to establish limits, prioritize projects, and stop squandering time. Effective time management facilitates your path of transformation and increases productivity.

9. Overcome Difficulties: Be prepared for setbacks and cultivate perseverance. Recognize that obstacles are an inherent feature of any process of change. Take lessons from your mistakes, adjust, and keep going.

10. Develop a Positive Attitude: Maintaining change requires a positive perspective. Refute pessimistic ideas, express thanks, and concentrate on your accomplishments.

11. Honor accomplishments: Give thanks and acknowledge minor setbacks along the route. Acknowledging your progress increases motivation and supports the constructive adjustments you are making. Recall that you are on a continuous path of transformation and that every step you take will bring you one step closer to living the life you have always desired.

CHAPTER FOUR

PERIODIC FASTING

Periodic Fasting Recent years have seen a considerable increase in interest in intermittent fasting (IF), a well-liked dietary strategy with possible health advantages beyond weight control.

This eating pattern revolves around eating and fasting in cycles, paying attention to both the timing and content of meals. Although the idea of fasting is not new, intermittent fasting (IF) has gained popularity due to its ease of use and its benefits for weight reduction, metabolism, and general health.

The flexibility of intermittent fasting is one of its main draws. Instead of dictating what you eat or how many calories you may consume, intermittent fasting (IF) focuses on when you should eat. The 16/8 approach, which calls for a 16-hour fast and an 8-hour eating window each day, and the 5:2 method, which permits regular eating five days a week but caps calorie intake at 500–600 on two non-consecutive days, are popular IF techniques.

The effect of intermittent fasting on insulin sensitivity is one of the main causes underlying it. Decrease insulin levels during fasting periods, improve blood sugar regulation, and decrease the likelihood of insulin resistance. Increased insulin sensitivity may be especially helpful for those who already have type 2 diabetes or are at risk of getting it. Studies indicate that fasting on and off could improve glycemic control and serve as an additional strategy for controlling blood sugar levels. In addition to its impact on insulin, intermittent fasting has been linked to a number of advantages for metabolism. The body switches from using glucose as its main energy source during fasting periods to using stored fat. This metabolic shift may result in more fat being burned, which would then cause weight reduction. For people trying to lose weight, intermittent fasting is a compelling alternative since some studies indicate it may be just as effective at managing weight as rigorous calorie restriction.

Moreover, there could be advantages for cardiovascular health from intermittent fasting. According to research, it may lower blood pressure, cholesterol, and triglycerides, among other cardiovascular risk factors. Heart disease continues to be the world's biggest cause of death; these advancements may help reduce the risk of heart disease. It's crucial to remember that everyone reacts differently to intermittent fasting, and more study is required to completely comprehend its long-term effects on cardiovascular health. Intermittent fasting has also been linked to cognitive advantages.

According to some research, fasting intervals may increase the body's synthesis of BDNF, a protein essential for memory, learning, and cognitive function. Furthermore, because oxidative stress and inflammation are linked to neurodegenerative disorders, intermittent fasting may promote brain health by lowering these two factors. Even though intermittent fasting has many potential health advantages, not everyone is a good match for it.

Before beginning an intermittent fast, people with specific medical issues, women who are pregnant or nursing, and those who have a history of eating disorders should exercise caution and speak with healthcare providers. It is important to stress that a nutrient-dense, well-balanced diet should be the main emphasis during eating periods while using intermittent fasting. A frequent misperception is that IF gives you permission to overindulge in junk food during your eating window. However, a well-rounded diet full of fruits, vegetables, lean meats, and whole grains must be prioritized for the best possible health results.

CHAPTER FIVE

DIET THAT REDUCES INFLAMMATION

Diet that Reduces Inflammation because anti-inflammatory diets lower inflammation in the body, they are essential for boosting general health and well-being. Although persistent inflammation may cause a number of health problems, such as diabetes, autoimmune disorders, and cardiovascular illnesses, it is a normal reaction to damage or infection. A healthy lifestyle may be promoted, and these risks can be reduced by using an anti-inflammatory diet.

Knowing About Inflammation: The body uses inflammation as a defensive mechanism when faced with dangerous stimuli like infections, damaged cells, or irritants. To defend and restore tissues, the immune system releases chemicals and white blood cells. On the other hand, persistent inflammation may cause long-term harm and be a factor in a number of chronic illnesses.

Nutrition's Function: Inflammation regulation is greatly influenced by nutrition. Certain meals have the ability to reduce or eliminate inflammation. The goal of an anti-inflammatory diet is to include foods that reduce inflammation while avoiding those that do the opposite.

IMPORTANT INGREDIENTS IN AN ANTI-INFLAMMATORY DIET

1. Omega-3 Fatty Acids: Rich in fatty fish such as salmon and mackerel, chia seeds also contain omega-3 fatty acids, which have strong anti-inflammatory properties. They lessen inflammation by assisting in the body's omega-3-to-omega-6 ratio balance.

2. Fruits and Vegetables: Intensely anti-inflammatory antioxidants and phytochemicals abound in colorful fruits and vegetables. In particular, cruciferous veggies like broccoli, leafy greens, and berries are healthy.

3. Whole Grains: Whole grains provide fiber and other nutrients that help to reduce inflammation. Examples of these are brown rice, quinoa, and oats. They also aid in blood sugar stabilization, which lowers the chance of inflammation.

 4. Nuts and Seeds: Rich in fiber, antioxidants, and good fats, nuts and seeds are a great source of nutrition. Nuts such as almonds, walnuts, flaxseeds, and chia seeds may be included in a regular diet.

5. Spices and Herbs: Anti-inflammatory qualities may be found in turmeric, ginger, garlic, and cinnamon. These spices provide health advantages in addition to adding taste to food.

6. Good Fats: Monounsaturated fats, such as those found in avocados, olive oils, and coconut oils, have anti-inflammatory properties. Additionally beneficial to general health and heart health are these lipids.

7. Probiotics: Fermented foods such as kefir, sauerkraut, and yogurt contain probiotics that help maintain a balanced micro biota in the stomach. Maintaining immunological function and controlling inflammation require a well-balanced gut micro biota.

SNACKS TO AVOID

1. Processed Foods: Processed foods often include high concentrations of harmful fats, refined sugars, and additives that may aggravate inflammation. Steer clear of them to improve your general health.

2. Highly Refined Carbohydrates: In an anti-inflammatory diet, foods with a high glycerin index, including white bread and sugary snacks, should be avoided since they may cause inflammation.

4. Overindulgence in Red Meat: Although lean meats may be included in a balanced diet, consuming too much red and processed meat can aggravate inflammation. Choosing protein sources derived from plants may be a healthier option.

A LIFE'S POSSIBILITIES

Inflammation is influenced by a few lifestyle choices in addition to food modifications. A healthy lifestyle that reduces inflammation includes regular exercise, getting enough sleep, managing stress, and quitting smoking.

THE FISCHER'S BASIS

An abundance of scientific research substantiates the beneficial effects of an anti-inflammatory diet on well-being. As an example, research that appeared in the "American Journal of Clinical Nutrition" showed that a diet high in fruits, vegetables, and whole grains was linked to a reduction in blood levels of inflammatory markers. The anti-inflammatory properties of omega-3 fatty acids, which are present in fish, have been the subject of much research. These fatty acids may help prevent and treat inflammatory diseases like rheumatoid arthritis since research indicates that they may regulate the inflammatory response.

STARTING A DIETARY ANTI-INFLAMMATORY

A gradual and persistent shift toward an anti-inflammatory diet is required. Increase the amount of fruits, vegetables, and whole grains that you eat. Try varying the herbs and spices to add flavor without using too much sugar or salt. One useful tactic to guarantee a varied and balanced diet is meal planning. Meal preparation at home gives you more control over the components, which makes it simpler to stay away from processed and inflammatory foods.

POSSIBLE ADVANTAGES:

1. Heart Health: A diet low in inflammation is linked to a lower risk of heart disease. Antioxidants and omega-3 fatty acids contribute to cardiovascular health.

2. Joint Health: An anti-inflammatory diet may provide treatment for those with inflammatory joint disorders such as arthritis. Certain foods have shown potential in the management of joint inflammation, including turmeric and fatty fish.

3. Weight control: Eating a diet low in inflammation may help with weight control. Placing focus on whole, nutrient-dense meals may aid in controlling hunger and averting overindulgence.

4. Better Gut Health: Consuming foods high in fiber and probiotics helps maintain a healthy gut flora, which is critical for boosting immunity and lowering inflammation.

CHAPTER SIX

FUEL REFOCUS

Encourage a Refocus The concept of "fuel refocus," which includes a wide range of programs meant to shift our energy use toward more ecologically friendly and sustainable sources, is important and topical. Global awareness of the need to replace our dependence on conventional fuels with alternative and renewable energy sources has grown in response to climate change and the depletion of fossil fuel supplies.

This shift in attention to fuel is not only required but also a step toward a more sustainable future. Shifting from fossil fuels like coal, oil, and natural gas to renewable energy sources like solar, wind, hydro, and geothermal energy is a crucial component of fuel emphasis. Burning fossil fuels has a well-documented negative environmental effect, greatly increasing air pollution and greenhouse gas emissions. We can lessen the negative consequences of climate change and lower our carbon footprint by shifting our attention back to renewable energy.

Among renewable energy sources, solar energy is a clear leader. The process of using solar panels to capture sunlight has become more economical and efficient. The likelihood that solar energy will provide a significant amount of our energy demands is increasing as technology develops. Globally, companies and governments are investing in solar infrastructure, and the move to solar energy is an important part of the fuel refocus agenda.

Another important component in the switch to renewable energy is wind power. When erected in locations with steady wind patterns, wind turbines provide power without emitting any hazardous gases. Wind energy may be used in both large-scale power plants and smaller, dispersed facilities due to its scalability. Its standing in the worldwide movement for sustainable energy solutions is further reinforced by the continuous innovation in wind turbine technology. For many years, hydropower—which is produced by the force of flowing water—has been a conventional renewable energy source. Water infrastructure, such as dams, uses the kinetic energy of flowing rivers to produce power. Large-scale dam construction raises environmental concerns; however, there are more ecologically acceptable options thanks to developments in low-impact hydropower technology.

Fuel refocus is a complex strategy that includes the creation of creative ideas and the optimization of current hydropower plants. To generate power and heat buildings, geothermal energy uses the heat that naturally exists inside the earth. It has the capacity to produce electricity continuously and is a dependable and steady power source.

The environmental impact of geothermal power stations is lower than that of conventional fossil fuel facilities. Geothermal energy is becoming more and more possible to integrate into the world's energy mix as technological advances make it more affordable and accessible. Fuel emphasis includes switching to renewable energy sources as well as increasing energy efficiency in a variety of industries. Transportation, industrial activities, and domestic energy usage are all examples of this. The use of electric vehicles (EVs) as a greener substitute for conventional gasoline-powered automobiles has grown.

Automakers are substantially investing in research and development to improve battery technology and boost the range of electric cars, while governments are providing incentives for the adoption of EVs. The industrial sector is looking for methods to streamline operations and cut down on energy waste since it accounts for a significant amount of the world's energy usage.

The overarching objective of reducing the environmental impact of industrial operations is aided by innovations like smart manufacturing, energy-efficient technology, and sustainable activities. Energy-efficient appliances, smart home technology, and better insulation techniques are important factors in lowering energy use at the household level. Incentives for energy-efficient modifications are often provided by governments and utility providers to homes, encouraging a more conscientious and sustainable fuel usage strategy. To sum up, fuel refocus is a comprehensive strategy that includes optimizing energy efficiency across several industries and shifting from fossil fuels to renewable energy sources. Adopting cleaner and more sustainable alternatives is crucial because of the pressing need to address climate change and the limited supply of fossil fuels.

The international community can together strive towards a future where our energy demands are satisfied in an ecologically friendly way via technological innovation, legislative efforts, and individual acts. The continuous effort to fuel refocus is a step toward a world that is more robust and sustainable.

CHAPTER SEVEN

THE NUTRITIONAL BASIS FOR THE GALVESTON DIET

The Galveston diet is a dietary strategy that emphasizes hormonal balance and the decrease of inflammation in order to promote women's health. This diet, developed by obstetrician-gynecologist Dr. Mary Claire Haver, places a strong emphasis on a holistic approach to health. The Galveston Diet is centered on certain dietary guidelines, lifestyle adjustments, and an awareness of how dietary decisions may affect hormonal health. The Galveston Diet has a strong focus on eating a diet low in carbohydrates, rich in healthy fats, and moderate in protein.

The objective is to control insulin sensitivity and blood sugar levels, two essential components of hormone regulation. The diet seeks to provide a stable metabolic environment by giving preference to foods that have little effect on blood sugar, such as leafy greens, non-starchy vegetables, and healthy fats like avocados and olive oil. Anti-inflammatory food intake is also encouraged by the dietary basis of the Galveston Diet.

Hormonal abnormalities are among the health problems that have been associated with chronic inflammation. Omega-3 fatty acid-rich foods, such as walnuts and fatty fish (salmon, mackerel), are marketed as having anti-inflammatory qualities. Furthermore, antioxidant-rich fruits and vegetables are essential for reducing inflammation.

The Galveston Diet's protein sources are selected for their favorable effects on hormones. Fish, chicken, and plant-based substitutes like tofu are good sources of lean protein as they are low in saturated fat and high in important amino acids. For the purposes of sustaining muscle mass, boosting metabolism, and encouraging satiety, an adequate protein intake is essential. The Galveston Diet prioritizes complex, high-fiber foods above simple sweets when it comes to carbs. Legumes, fiber-rich vegetables, and whole grains all help maintain steady energy levels and prevent sharp increases in blood sugar. This strategy supports the main objective of the diet, which is to maintain hormonal balance by minimizing insulin swings.

Another element included in the Galveston Diet is intermittent fasting. Periods of fasting are thought to benefit weight control, increase autophagy (cellular repair), and improve insulin sensitivity. The diet usually includes a window of time each day for fasting, during which the only foods allowed are water, herbal tea, and black coffee. Additionally acknowledging the significance of gut health for general well-being is the Galveston Diet.

It is advised to consume fermented foods such as sauerkraut, kefir, and yogurt to support a balanced population of good gut bacteria. Improved immunological response, emotional modulation, and digestion have all been related to a healthy gut flora. On the Galveston Diet, supplements are sometimes advised to treat certain vitamin shortages. Individual requirements may dictate the use of some supplements, such as magnesium, vitamin D, and omega-3 fatty acids. The goal of these supplements is to enhance general health and support the focus on hormonal balance in the diet.

The Galveston Diet stresses lifestyle aspects that support hormonal health in addition to nutritional recommendations. Regular physical exercise, stress reduction, and enough sleep are seen as essential elements of the whole strategy. Hormone control, especially cortisol and growth hormone, depends on sleep. Cortisol regulation involves the use of stress-reduction strategies like mindfulness and meditation. It is advised to exercise, particularly strength and cardiovascular training, to promote metabolic health and preserve muscle mass.

Exercise enhances general health and supports the goals of the diet by fostering hormonal balance.

CHAPTER EIGHT

PUTTING IT ALL TOGETHER. THE MEAL PLANS AND SHOPPING LISTS

Combining everything To build a simplified and effective approach to nutrition and grocery shopping, it all comes down to smoothly combining shopping lists and meal planning. Careful meal preparation is essential to a successful health-conscious practice since it guarantees a balance of nutrients, tastes, and variation. Concurrently, a well-designed shopping list becomes the essential instrument for making these goals a reality.

Weekly meal plans are like a template for how much food should be consumed. They provide a planned framework for daily meals by accounting for dietary choices, nutritional objectives, and culinary tastes. The proper ratios of proteins, carbs, fats, vitamins, and minerals are carefully considered while planning breakfasts, lunches, dinners, and snacks. This deliberate preparation not only improves general health but also deters impulsive and harmful eating decisions.

When you have a meal plan in place, the shopping list becomes your constant partner. It turns the theoretical concept of a well-rounded diet into concrete products that can be purchased at the grocery store. A well-structured shopping list divides things into categories according to store departments, making shopping easier and reducing the likelihood of missing necessary supplies. One useful way to make a grocery list is to make sure all the ingredients are included by comparing it to the meals that are scheduled.

This contributes to cost-effectiveness and environmental sustainability by reducing the need for frequent grocery visits and food waste. Technology integration may improve this procedure even further. Making and maintaining grocery lists and meal plans may be done more effectively by using digital platforms or applications for meal planning. These instruments often provide effortless adjustment, offering adaptability for evolving dietary requirements or inclinations.

CHAPTER NINE

DIET OF GALVESTON RECIPES

Galveston Diet Recipes Dr. Mary Claire Haver created the Galveston Diet, which emphasizes hormonal balance, especially for menopausal women. The Galveston diet doesn't have a set of official recipes, even though it stresses eating healthily. Rather, it advocates for a nutritionally balanced diet that includes a range of whole foods.

The Galveston diet has a strong focus on anti-inflammatory foods. A wide variety of vibrant vegetables, lean meats like fish and chicken, and healthy fats like avocados and olive oil are often included in recipes. These components are intended to promote general well-being and reduce inflammation, which might worsen during menopause.

A sample meal for the Galveston diet may be grilled fish along with roasted vegetables that have been spiced with anti-inflammatory herbs like ginger and turmeric. Nuts, seeds, and leafy greens are often included in salads, which provide a filling and nutrient-dense meal.

The diet promotes a more sustainable and well-balanced way of eating by discouraging processed foods, refined sugars, and an abundance of carbs. Beyond only offering recipes, Dr. Haver's philosophy encourages people to make decisions that support their overall health objectives. It's crucial to remember that people should speak with a healthcare provider before making big dietary changes, particularly if they have underlying medical issues.

Although there isn't a rigid set of recipes associated with the Galveston diet, its tenets may direct people toward a more nutritious and well-rounded approach to eating after menopause.

CHAPTER TEN

DIET OF GALVESTON FOR LIFE

The Lifelong Galveston Diet As a lifestyle approach to diet that emphasizes total health and well-being above weight reduction, the Galveston Diet has grown in popularity. This diet plan was created by OB-GYN Dr. Mary Claire Haver, who has a strong interest in women's health. It is intended to help women with the particular difficulties they have in reaching and maintaining a healthy weight.

The main goal of the Galveston Diet is to lessen internal inflammation. While the body naturally responds to inflammation as a means of healing, persistent inflammation may cause a number of health problems, including weight gain. Dr. Haver's methods include reducing or removing inflammatory items from the diet and increasing anti-inflammatory ones.

The Galveston Diet has a strong focus on entire, nutrient-dense meals. Fruits, vegetables, lean meats, and good fats are some of them. The Galveston Diet's recommended foods are high in antioxidants, vitamins, and minerals, with the goal of promoting general health and decreasing inflammation.

The diet also promotes intermittent fasting, which involves alternating between eating and fasting intervals. Numerous health advantages, such as better weight control and insulin sensitivity, have been associated with this strategy. A 16:8 fasting window, in which people fast for 16 hours and eat for 8 hours, is what Dr. Haver suggests.

The Galveston Diet is unique in that it takes into account women's hormonal changes. Dr. Haver agrees that fluctuations in hormones, especially in perimenopause and menopause, might affect metabolism and weight. Because of this, the diet has particular suggestions to assist hormonal balance, such as consuming foods high in phytoestrogens and controlling stress levels. The Galveston Diet emphasizes proper sleep and frequent exercise in addition to nutritional recommendations. Engaging in physical exercise enhances general wellbeing in addition to helping with weight control. In a similar vein, getting enough good sleep is critical for maintaining hormone balance and general wellness.

The adaptability of the Galveston Diet is one of its advantages. It may be tailored to accommodate a broad variety of dietary requirements, such as being gluten-free or vegetarian. This flexibility helps the diet remain sustainable over time as a way of life option rather than a temporary fix.

Although a lot of people who follow the Galveston Diet claim success, it's important to remember that everyone reacts differently to different dietary methods. Before making big dietary changes, it is advised that people speak with healthcare providers, particularly if they have underlying medical issues.